MW01247336

WEIGHT WATCHERS

THE SMART POINTS COOKBOOK

FOR BEGINNERS

30 Days Weight Watchers Meal Plan

With 40+ Quick and Easy Recipes

James Houck

COPYRIGHT 2016 - ALL RIGHTS RESERVED

CONTENTS

1   Introduction to Weight Watchers   Pg. 4

2   History of Weight Watchers   Pg. 5

3   Weight Watchers: Smart Points   Pg. 6

4   Pros and Cons of Smart Points   Pg. 7

5   Smart Points Calculator   Pg. 9

6   30 Days Smart Points Meal Plan   Pg. 10

7   Breakfast, Lunch, and Dinner Recipes   Pg. 14

8   Breakfast Recipes   Pg. 14

9   Lunch Recipes   Pg. 31

10 Dinner Recipes   Pg. 46

11 About the Author   Pg. 62

INTRODUCTION TO WEIGHT WATCHERS

Weight Watchers is not just a regular diet; it's a lifestyle. Weight Watchers is about people making healthier food choices for a happier life.

The Weight Watchers philosophy is really simple. It focuses on adopting a sensible approach centered on achieving and maintaining a healthy weight by adopting a sensible approach of making wiser food choices and moving towards positive behavioral changes.

Weight Watchers is not an advocate of quick fix weight loss or fad diets. It is a well-established program that can achieve lasting results.

HISTORY OF WEIGHT WATCHERS

It all began when a 214-pound housewife, Jean Nidetch, got discouraged by many years of fad dieting. In desperation to lose weight, Jean attended a free diet clinic and was able to lose 20 pounds, but then her motivation started waning.

It's then when she picked up her phone and made her cookie confession to a few of her overweight friends. Her friends not only understood what Jean was going through but shared their confessions as well. After that, these women started coming to Jean's house on weekly basis for mutual support and sharing.

Interestingly, they all lost weight and, together, they realized that weight loss is more than just following a diet. It's all about changing old habits and getting support and encouragement from people who care for you and, thus, WEIGHT WATCHERS established as a company in May 1963.

WEIGHT WATCHERS: SMART POINTS

In 2016, Weight Watchers announced that they are moving to a new program, "Beyond The Scale" and with that the points system will also change. Weight Watchers is moving from the old points system of Points Plus to a new and healthier points system, "Smart Points".

Smart Points is a much easier and simpler counting system to use. Smart Points pushes you towards healthier, nutritious foods so that you eat and feel better, gain more energy and, most importantly, lose weight. Now, that's what I call SMART!

With Smart Points, food items that are higher in saturated fat and/or sugar are higher in Smart Points values. Food items that have high lean protein are scored lower in Smart Points values. As you can see, you are directed towards healthier choices.

- Every food is allocated its own Smart Points value based on four components: saturated fat, calories, protein, and sugar.

- Protein lowers the Smart Points values.

- Sugar and saturated fat surge the Smart Points values.

In nutshell, it rewards you for eating less sugar and saturated fat, and more lean protein.

Another important change in the new point systems is that FitPoints® have replaced Activity Points and the new points are calculated based on different kinds of activities ranging from daily chores to more planned exercise.

Under the Points Plus approach, you were given 49 weekly points to use however you wanted. In the Smart Points approach, this number will be adjusted based on your weight loss goals, activity level, gender, age, and other factors.

PROS AND CONS OF SMART POINTS

As you know any new system has its pros and cons and it's really important for you to be aware of both so that you can take informed decision. Let's take a look at some of the pros and cons of using the new Smart Points approach:

Pros

- Smart Points main objective is to close all the loopholes that exist within the Points Plus approach. For example, the Point Plus approach use to encourage people to eat foods that are loaded with sugars and other additives. This made them taste as good as full fat foods.

- Under the Point Plus approach, if you are doing exercise, you can earn more points that you can spend on food. In nutshell, if you want to eat more, exercise more. This lead to unhealthy mindset about food and how it should be used to fuel your body. Under the new Smart Points approach, you can no longer trade your exercise points with food. In nutshell, the new system separates your food intake and the activity.

- The new Smart Points system is more about creating overall healthier lifestyle and less about weight loss. Whereas, the Points Plus system use to focus on counting calories. The Smart Points encourages you to choose the foods with the least sugar and most protein, which is a healthier choice for a healthier lifestyle.

Cons

- For many experienced Weight Watchers, the biggest drawback is to get used to the new system, especially, when they have enjoyed success with Points Plus. These members can still use the Points Plus system, but to be honest, Weight Watchers will definitely phase it out.

- Many people claim that the Points Plus use to provide them amazing freedom and flexibility, which might not be the case with Smart Points as it pushes some of the foods away for the others.

- Eating sugar and saturated fat will have higher penalties than the Points Plus system. Some Weight Watchers members believe that the penalties for cookies and cake are now so high that it might cause some members to go off-plan and eat the foods that might affect their will power.

SMART POINTS CALCULATOR

It's worthwhile to note that over 50% of the Points Plus points will be changed when you move to Smart Points. Foods with lean proteins will quickly lower your points value. You will also love the fact that now lean meats, for example, prawns, turkey, and most seafood will have just 1 Smart Points, while chicken will drop to just 2 Smart Points (which use to worth 3 Points Plus earlier).

Points on dairy products have gone up even if it's 'non-fat' or 'low-fat'. Sugar is also a strictly no-n0 area as, now, one tablespoon of granulated white sugar will have up to 3 Smart Points which use to be 1 under the Points Plus approach. This will be huge change for people who like a piece of chocolate or sugar in their tea.

Fruits and vegetables will remain point-free but with one important change: fruits included in other recipes will now be free too.

Here is the rough Smart Points food value calculation:

(Calories * .0305) + (Sat Fat * .275) + (Sugar * .12) - (Protein * .098)

For example, if a food item has the following nutritional value:

Calories; 330, Protein 2g, Carbs 70g, Fibre 0g, Total Fat 5g, Saturated Fat 3g, and sugar 57g

The Smart Points value would be:

(330 cal * .0305) + (3g fat * .275) + (57g sugar * .12) - (2g Protein * .098) = **18 smart points**

30 DAYS SMART POINTS MEAL PLAN

Under the new plan, most people will find that they are allowed more Smart Points daily. The minimum daily points target is now **30 Smart Points** so anyone under 30 daily points will now have more.

The table below is a sample meal plan of a 5'2", 133lb female with a medium activity. This does not include snacks or FitPoints. You can use the balance points, after deducting the total points per day from 30 Smart Points.

Please note that each person's allowance is individual and is not a set calculation. This is also true of the weekly allowance as well. You will find detailed recipes followed by the meal plan. I have provided more recipes than listed in the plan below. So, feel free to swap recipes as per your taste and convenience.

	Breakfast	Smart Points	Lunch	Smart Points	Dinner	Smart Points	Total Points
DAY 1	Baked Italian Eggs	5	Salisbury Steak	5	BLT Pasta Salad	7	**17**
DAY 2	Potato Cutlet	7	Salsa Chicken	4	Chicken and Cheese Casserole	5	**16**
DAY 3	Breakfast Egg-Topped Hash	6	Tuna Salad	3	Quick Chili	7	**16**
DAY 4	French Omelet	3	Chicken and Dumplings	4	Barbecue Meatloaf	7	**14**
DAY 5	Potato Cutlet	7	Lemon and Herb Shrimp	2	Jalapeno Chicken	5	**14**
DAY 6	Banana Bread Overnight Oats	7	Baked Chicken with Lemon	2	Chicken Noodle Soup	5	**14**
DAY 7	Banana Smoothie	5	Parmesan Chicken Cutlets	3	Balsamic Chicken	5	**13**

	Breakfast	Smart Points	Lunch	Smart Points	Dinner	Smart Points	Total Points
DAY 8	Applesauce Oatmeal with Cranberry	5	Lemon Garlic Scallops	3	Crumbed Baked Chicken	5	**13**
DAY 9	Baked Italian Eggs	5	Lemon Pepper Chicken	3	Tuna Pasta Salad	5	**13**
DAY 10	Green Omelet	6	Turkey Sausage with Bell Peppers	3	Cilantro and Lime Shrimp	3	**12**
DAY 11	French Toast	3	Turkey Meatballs	4	Tuna Pasta Salad	5	**12**
DAY 12	French Toast	3	Egg Drop Chicken Soup	3	Crockpot Chicken Chili	5	**11**
DAY 13	French Omelet	3	Cheesy Eggplant Casserole	4	Chicken Salad	4	**11**
DAY 14	French Toast	3	Cola Chicken	5	Egg salad	3	**11**
DAY 15	Super Cherry-Vanilla Yogurt	5	Chicken Fried Rice	4	Stir Fried Chinese Vegetables	1	**10**

	Breakfast	Smart Points	Lunch	Smart Points	Dinner	Smart Points	Total Points
DAY 16	Baked Italian Eggs	5	Salisbury Steak	5	BLT Pasta Salad	7	**17**
DAY 17	Potato Cutlet	7	Salsa Chicken	4	Chicken and Cheese Casserole	5	**16**
DAY 18	Breakfast Egg-Topped Hash	6	Tuna Salad	3	Quick Chili	7	**16**
DAY 19	French Omelet	3	Chicken and Dumplings	4	Barbecue Meatloaf	7	**14**
DAY 20	Potato Cutlet	7	Lemon and Herb Shrimp	2	Jalapeno Chicken	5	**14**
DAY 21	Banana Bread Overnight Oats	7	Baked Chicken with Lemon	2	Chicken Noodle Soup	5	**14**
DAY 22	Banana Smoothie	5	Parmesan Chicken Cutlets	3	Balsamic Chicken	5	**13**

	Breakfast	Smart Points	Lunch	Smart Points	Dinner	Smart Points	Total Points
DAY 23	Applesauce Oatmeal with Cranberry	5	Lemon Garlic Scallops	3	Crumbed Baked Chicken	5	**13**
DAY 24	Baked Italian Eggs	5	Lemon Pepper Chicken	3	Tuna Pasta Salad	5	**13**
DAY 25	Green Omelet	6	Turkey Sausage with Bell Peppers	3	Cilantro and Lime Shrimp	3	**12**
DAY 26	French Toast	3	Turkey Meatballs	4	Tuna Pasta Salad	5	**12**
DAY 27	French Toast	3	Egg Drop Chicken Soup	3	Crockpot Chicken Chili	5	**11**
DAY 28	French Omelet	3	Cheesy Eggplant Casserole	4	Chicken Salad	4	**11**
DAY 29	French Toast	3	Cola Chicken	5	Egg salad	3	**11**
DAY 30	Super Cherry-Vanilla Yogurt	5	Chicken Fried Rice	4	Stir Fried Chinese Vegetables	1	**10**

BREAKFAST, LUNCH, & DINNER RECIPES

BREAKFAST RECIPES

POTATO CUTLET

SERVING SIZE: 1
SERVINGS PER RECIPE: 4
SMART POINTS PER SERVING: 7
CALORIES: 108
PREPARATION TIME: 10 MINUTES
INGREDIENTS:
1. 5 potatoes
2. 2 tbsp. salt
3. 6 tbsp. bread crumbs
4. Cooking oil
5. 10 cilantro leaves

NUTRITION INFORMATION

Fat	30g
Saturated Fat	24g
Carbohydrates	3g
Protein	26g
Sugar	0g

INSTRUCTIONS:
1. Cook the potatoes in the boiling water until they become tender and soft.
2. Cool, drain, and peel the potatoes.
3. Fry the potatoes in oil until the golden brown color and add all the ingredients mentioned above.

FRENCH OMELET

SERVING SIZE: 1
SERVINGS PER RECIPE: 4
SMART POINTS PER SERVING: 3
CALORIES: 154
PREPARATION TIME: 10 MINUTES
INGREDIENTS:
1. 2 eggs
2. 2 tbsp. water
3. 2 tbsp. salt
4. Dash pepper
5. 1/3 cup of shredded cheese

NUTRITION INFORMATION

Fat	12g
Saturated Fat	3.3g
Carbohydrates	0.6g
Protein	11g
Sugar	0g

INSTRUCTIONS:
1. Beat eggs, water salt, pepper until the mixture is blended.
2. Heat the pan with butter and pour the mixture onto it.
3. When you don't see the liquid egg mixture, gently fold the omelet in half and slide it into a plate.

FRENCH TOAST

SERVING SIZE: 1
SERVINGS PER RECIPE: 4
SMART POINTS PER SERVING: 3
CALORIES: 229
PREPARATION TIME: 10 MINUTES
INGREDIENTS:
1. 1 egg
2. 1 tbsp. vanilla extract
3. ½ tbsp. cinnamon
4. ¼ cup milk
5. 4 slices of bread

NUTRITION INFORMATION

Fat	11g
Saturated Fat	2.7g
Carbohydrates	25g
Protein	8g
Sugar	0g

INSTRUCTIONS:
1. Beat egg, vanilla, and cinnamon in shallow dish. Stir in milk.
2. Dip bread in egg mixture to be coated both sides evenly.
3. Cook bread slices on a skillet or lightly-greased nonstick griddle on medium heat until they are browned on both sides.

BANANA SMOOTHIE

SERVING SIZE: 1
SERVINGS PER RECIPE: 4
SMART POINTS PER SERVING: 5
CALORIES: 160
PREPARATION TIME: 10 MINUTES
INGREDIENTS:

1. 4 tbsp. blanched and de-skinned almonds
2. 1 cup bananas
3. 1 1/2 cups milk
4. 2 tbsp. sugar
5. 1/2 tbsp. vanilla essence
6. Ice-cubes

NUTRITION INFORMATION

Fat	10g
Saturated Fat	0g
Carbohydrates	0g
Protein	11g
Sugar	11g

INSTRUCTIONS:

1. Combine the bananas, almonds, and ½ cup of milk; and blend them in a juicer till the mixture is frothy and smooth.
2. Add the sugar, remaining 1 cup of milk, vanilla essence, and 8 ice cubes.
3. Blend in a juicer till the mixture is frothy and smooth.
4. Pour equal quantities of the smoothie into 4 individual glasses.

BURRITOS IN BREAKFAST

SERVING SIZE: 1
SERVINGS PER RECIPE: 4
SMART POINTS PER SERVING: 9
CALORIES: 298
PREPARATION TIME: 30 MINUTES
INGREDIENTS:

1. 2 teaspoon of olive oil
2. 2 chopped scallion
3. 1 chopped tomato
4. 1 chopped green pepper
5. 2 minced clove garlic
6. 2 eggs whole
7. 4 egg white
8. ½ cup shredded low-fat cheddar cheese
9. 2 tbsp. chopped cilantro
10. ¼ teaspoon salt and pepper
11. 4 whole wheat tortillas
12. ½ cup nonfat sour cream
13. ½ cup salsa

NUTRITION INFORMATION

Fat	9g
Saturated Fat	2g
Carbohydrates	37g
Protein	17g
Sugar	5g

INSTRUCTIONS:
1. Grease a baking dish with oil or non-stick cooking spray and preheat the oven to 400 degrees F.
2. Heat olive oil and then add scallions, green pepper, garlic, tomato and sauté. Let them get cook for 5 min. While cooking, stir in whole eggs and egg whites and then cook till you feel like it is cooked. Stop the stove and add in cheddar cheese, cilantro, pepper, and salt.
3. Place the tortilla in the baking dish and add the fillings before rolling the burritos.
4. Bake for 10 minutes and serve easily with sour cream and salsa.

APPLE PANCAKES WITH CINNAMON

SERVING SIZE: 1
SERVINGS PER RECIPE: 2
SMART POINTS PER SERVING: 5
CALORIES: 210
PREPARATION TIME: 20 MINUTES
INGREDIENTS:
1. ¾ cup of whole wheat flour
2. ½ tablespoon baking powder
3. 2 tbsp. sugar substitute
4. ½ tbsp. ground cinnamon
5. 1 cup water
6. 1 whole egg white lightly beaten
7. 1/3 cup applesauce, unsweetened

NUTRITION INFORMATION

Fat	1g
Saturated Fat	0g
Carbohydrates	43g
Protein	11g
Sugar	0g

INSTRUCTIONS:
1. Combine whole wheat flour, cinnamon, sugar substitute, and baking powder in a bowl.
2. Take another bowl and mix water, applesauce, and egg white.
3. Stir both the mixtures together until there are no lumps.
4. Take a skillet and heat it. Spray non-stick cooking spray.
5. Spread the batter lightly over the skillet and cook until you see the reddish brown color on both sides.

APPLESAUCE OATMEAL WITH CRANBERRY

SERVING SIZE: 1
SERVINGS PER RECIPE: 1
SMART POINTS PER SERVING: 5
CALORIES: 111
PREPARATION TIME: 4 MINUTES
INGREDIENTS:

1. 3 tbsp. uncooked oatmeal
2. 1 tbsp. dried cranberry
3. ½ cup of applesauce, unsweetened
4. ½ cup water
5. 1/8 tbsp. ground cinnamon

NUTRITION INFORMATION

Fat	1g
Saturated Fat	0g
Carbohydrates	25g
Protein	2g
Sugar	12g

INSTRUCTIONS:

1. Take a bowl and mix oatmeal, cranberries, applesauce, water, and cinnamon
2. Microwave the mixture for 2 minutes.

BAKED ITALIAN EGGS

SERVING SIZE: 1
SERVINGS PER RECIPE: 4
SMART POINTS PER SERVING: 7
CALORIES: 215
PREPARATION TIME: 30 MINUTES
INGREDIENTS:
1. 2 cup marinara sauce
2. ¼ cup fresh basil
3. 4 large egg
4. ½ cup parmesan cheese

NUTRITION INFORMATION

Fat	8g
Saturated Fat	6g
Carbohydrates	29g
Protein	12g
Sugar	0g

INSTRUCTIONS:
1. Preheat the oven to 350 degrees F.
2. Pour marinara sauce in the skillet and sprinkle basil over. Make narrow wells and crack an egg into the center of each one. Sprinkle parmesan cheese over it.
3. Bake for 20 min.

SCRAMBLED GREEK EGG WRAPS

SERVING SIZE: 1
SERVINGS PER RECIPE: 2
SMART POINTS PER SERVING: 14
CALORIES: 383
PREPARATION TIME: 10 MINUTES
INGREDIENTS:
1. 1 small zucchini
2. 1 low-fat cooking spray
3. 8 cherry tomato
4. 1/2 red onion
5. 1/4 cup black olives, chopped (half a small can)
6. 1/2 cup reduced-fat feta cheese
7. 1 1/2 tbsp. (up to 2) Greek seasoning
8. 4 egg
9. 4 to 6 flour tortilla

NUTRITION INFORMATION

Fat	16g
Saturated Fat	5g
Carbohydrates	40g
Protein	19g
Sugar	6g

INSTRUCTIONS:

1. Spray a little cooking spray on a non-stick skillet pan.
2. Chop the red onion finely and set aside.
3. Shred/grate the zucchini and allow soaking of any moisture by laying the flesh on a paper towel.
4. Cut the cherry tomatoes quarterly, take out the seeds, and finely chop the flesh. Allow soaking of any moisture by laying the flesh on a paper towel.
5. Chop finely the feta cheese and the black olives. Set both aside, separately.
6. Beat the eggs with the Greek seasoning.
7. Saute the chopped onion in the non-stick skillet for 2 minutes over medium heat and stir.
8. Add the tomatoes, zucchini, and olives; and cook for another minute.
9. Add the beaten eggs and cook for another 3-4 minutes, but stir or until done.
10. Place some egg mixture on each wrap, and add the feta cheese at the top. Fold the wrap and enjoy!

BREAKFAST EGG-TOPPED HASH

SERVING SIZE: 1
SERVINGS PER RECIPE: 2
SMART POINTS PER SERVING: 6
CALORIES: 225
PREPARATION TIME: 10 MINUTES
INGREDIENTS:
1. 1 cup roughly chopped cauliflower
2. 1/4 cup quick-cooking corn grits
3. 2 dashes salt
4. 1/4 cup (about 2 large) egg whites
5. 1/4 cup shredded reduced-fat cheddar cheese
6. 3 cups roughly chopped spinach leaves
7. 1 tbsp. dried minced onion
8. 2 large eggs
9. Optional topping: black pepper

NUTRITION INFORMATION

Fat	8g
Saturated Fat	3.5g
Carbohydrates	21g
Protein	17g
Sugar	2.5g

INSTRUCTIONS:

1. Beat the cauliflower in a blender until it is reduced to rice-sized pieces. Then, transfer it to a microwave-safe bowl.
2. Add a dash of salt, grits, and 1/3 cup water and mix well. Cover the mixture and microwave it for 2 minutes, or until thickened.
3. Stir well and let it cool for 5 minutes.
4. Add cheese and egg whites, and mix thoroughly.
5. Bring a large skillet and spray it with nonstick spray at medium-high heat. Cook and beat the cauliflower mixture for about 6 minutes till it's fully cooked and lightly browned.
6. Add onion, spinach, and remaining dash of salt. Cook and stir for about 1 minute until spinach has blended.
7. Divide mixture between 2 bowls or plates, and cover it to keep warm.
8. Remove skillet from heat. Re-spray, after cleaning if needed, and bring it to medium heat. Crack eggs into the skillet and cook per your preference or cook one at a time.
9. Top each hash portion with an egg.

GREEN OMELET

SERVING SIZE: 1
SERVINGS PER RECIPE: 1
SMART POINTS PER SERVING: 6
CALORIES: 187
PREPARATION TIME: 10 MINUTES
INGREDIENTS:

1. 1 cup sliced mushrooms
2. 1/2 tbsp. chopped garlic
3. 1 cup frozen French-cut green beans
4. 2 cups chopped spinach leaves
5. 1 wedge The Laughing Cow Light Creamy Swiss cheese
6. 3/4 cup fat-free liquid egg substitute (like Egg Beaters Original)
7. Optional seasonings: salt and black pepper
8. Optional toppings: salsa verde, fat-free sour cream

NUTRITION INFORMATION

Fat	2g
Saturated Fat	1g
Carbohydrates	14.5g
Protein	25g
Sugar	6g

INSTRUCTIONS:

1. Bring a medium-sized skillet with a lid and spray it with nonstick spray at medium heat. Cook and stir garlic and mushrooms for about 4 minutes till they are slightly softened.

2. Add frozen green beans, and continue cooking for about 2 minutes until green beans are hot and mushrooms are soft. Add spinach, cook for about 1 minute, and stir until wilted.

3. Get a medium bowl, transfer veggies into it, and blot the excess moisture. Add cheese wedge, break it into pieces, and stir till it's distributed thoroughly. Cover it to keep warm.

4. Clean the skillet, if needed. Remove the skillet from heat, spray again, and return it on a medium heat. Then, add egg substitute, and let it rub the bottom of the skillet.

5. Cover and cook it for 3 minutes without stirring, or until just set.

6. Serve veggie mixture onto one half of the omelet. Fold the other half over the filling, and slide your stuffed omelet onto a plate!

SUPER CHERRY-VANILLA YOGURT

SERVING SIZE: 1
SERVINGS PER RECIPE: 1
SMART POINTS PER SERVING: 5
CALORIES: 268
PREPARATION TIME: 5 MINUTES
INGREDIENTS:
1. About ½ cup or one 5.3-oz. container fat-free plain Greek yogurt
2. 2 tbsp. vanilla protein powder (like the kind by Tera's Whey)
3. 2 tbsp. light vanilla soymilk, unsweetened vanilla almond milk, or fat-free dairy milk
4. Dash cinnamon
5. 1 1/2 tbsp. chia seeds
6. 3/4 cup chopped unsweetened dark pitted sweet cherries
7. 1/4 oz. (about 1 tbsp.) sliced almonds

NUTRITION INFORMATION

Fat	6.5g
Saturated Fat	.5g
Carbohydrates	29g
Protein	26.5g
Sugar	21g

INSTRUCTIONS:
1. In a medium jar, combine protein powder, yogurt, cinnamon, and milk. Mix until smooth and uniform. Stir in chia seeds.
2. Top with almonds and cherries, or stir them in.

BANANA BREAD OVERNIGHT OATS

SERVING SIZE: 1
SERVINGS PER RECIPE: 1
SMART POINTS PER SERVING: 7
CALORIES: 303
PREPARATION TIME: 5 MINUTES
INGREDIENTS:
1. 1/2 cup unsweetened vanilla almond milk
2. 1/4 cup fat-free plain Greek yogurt
3. 1 packet no-calorie sweetener (like Truvia)
4. 1/8 tbsp. cinnamon
5. 1/8 tbsp. vanilla extract
6. 1/8 tbsp. maple extract
7. Dash salt
8. 1/2 cup old-fashioned oats
9. 1/4 cup mashed extra-ripe banana
10. 1/4 oz. (about 1 tbsp.) chopped walnuts

NUTRITION INFORMATION

Fat	9g
Saturated Fat	1g
Carbohydrates	45g
Protein	13.5g
Sugar	10.5g

INSTRUCTIONS:
1. In a medium jar or bowl, combine yogurt, almond milk, sweetener, cinnamon, maple extract, vanilla extract, and salt. Mix until uniform.
2. Stir in banana and oats.
3. Cover and refrigerate 6 hours at least, until oats have absorbed the liquid and are soft.
4. Top with walnuts.

LUNCH RECIPES

LEMON AND HERB SHRIMP

SERVING SIZE: 1
SERVINGS PER RECIPE: 4
SMART POINTS PER SERVING: 2
CALORIES: 103
PREPARATION TIME: 15 MINUTES
INGREDIENTS:
1. 2 tbsp. olive oil
2. 1 lb large shrimp, peeled
3. 2 tbsp. lemon juice
4. 1 tbsp. salt-free lemon and herb seasoning
5. ½ tbsp. table salt
6. ¼ tbsp. black pepper
7. 2 tbsp. parsley

NUTRITION INFORMATION

Fat	3g
Saturated Fat	0g
Carbohydrates	2g
Protein	16g
Sugar	0g

INSTRUCTIONS:
1. Heat oil in a skillet and add shrimp and sauté. Cook for 1 min and add lemon juice, lemon herb seasoning, salt, and pepper; and stir.
2. Remove from heat and stir in parsley.

BAKED CHICKEN WITH LEMON

SERVING SIZE: 1
SERVINGS PER RECIPE: 4
SMART POINTS PER SERVING: 2
CALORIES: 146
PREPARATION TIME: 45 MINUTES
INGREDIENTS:
1. 1 lb boneless chicken
2. ½ tbsp. salt
3. 1/4 tbsp. black pepper and cup chicken broth
4. 1 tbsp. olive oil
5. 2 tbsp. fresh lemon juice, fresh rosemary, fresh parsley
6. 1 lemon

NUTRITION INFORMATION

Fat	4g
Saturated Fat	1g
Carbohydrates	1g
Protein	25g
Sugar	0g

INSTRUCTIONS:
1. Preheat the oven to 400 degrees F.
2. Season all sides of chicken with salt and black pepper. Take a pan and sprinkle with olive oil, place the chicken on the pan, sprinkle lemon juice, rosemary, and parsley and, pour broth around the chicken.
3. Bake for 35 minutes.

EGG DROP CHICKEN SOUP

SERVING SIZE: 1
SERVINGS PER RECIPE: 5
SMART POINTS PER SERVING: 3
CALORIES: 119
PREPARATION TIME: 10 MINUTES
INGREDIENTS:
1. 4 cup chicken broth
2. ½ tbsp. soy sauce
3. ½ cup cooked boneless chicken and frozen green peas
4. ¼ cup green onion
5. 1 egg

NUTRITION INFORMATION

Fat	4g
Saturated Fat	1g
Carbohydrates	8g
Protein	14g
Sugar	2g

INSTRUCTIONS:
1. Boil chicken stock and soy sauce in a saucepan. Add chicken, green onions, and peas. Boil again.
2. Stop heating and drizzle with egg in steady stream and wait 1 min for egg to set.

PARMESAN CHICKEN CUTLETS

SERVING SIZE: 1
SERVINGS PER RECIPE: 4
SMART POINTS PER SERVING: 3
CALORIES: 172
PREPARATION TIME: 35 MINUTES
INGREDIENTS:
1. ¼ cup parmesan cheese
2. 2 tbsp. seasoned bread crumbs
3. 1/8 tbsp. paprika
4. 1 tbsp. dried parsley
5. 1/2 tbsp. garlic powder
6. 1/4 tbsp. black pepper
7. 1 pound boneless chicken

NUTRITION INFORMATION

Fat	5g
Saturated Fat	2g
Carbohydrates	3g
Protein	27g
Sugar	0g

INSTRUCTIONS:
1. Preheat oven to 400 degrees F. Take a plastic bag and add cheese, crumbs, and seasonings and shake well.
2. Dip the chicken in the mixture properly and arrange on nonstick baking sheet.
3. Bake for 25 minutes.

LEMON GARLIC SCALLOPS

SERVING SIZE: 1
SERVINGS PER RECIPE: 4
SMART POINTS PER SERVING: 3
CALORIES: 151
PREPARATION TIME: 15 MINUTES
INGREDIENTS:

1. 1 tbsp. olive oil
2. 1 ¼ lb sea scallop
3. 2 tbsp. all-purpose flour and parsley
4. ¼ tbsp. salt
5. 6 garlic cloves
6. 1 scallion
7. 1 pinch sage
8. 1 lemon, juiced

NUTRITION INFORMATION

Fat	4g
Saturated Fat	1g
Carbohydrates	10g
Protein	18g
Sugar	0g

INSTRUCTIONS:

1. Heat oil in a large skillet. In a bowl, mix scallops, flour, and salt.
2. Place scallops on the skillet; add garlic, scallions, and sage.
3. Sauté for 4 min and stir in lemon juice and parsley. Serve immediately.

LEMON PEPPER CHICKEN

SERVING SIZE: 1
SERVINGS PER RECIPE: 4
SMART POINTS PER SERVING: 3
CALORIES: 139
PREPARATION TIME: 35 MINUTES
INGREDIENTS:
1. 2 tbsp. lemon pepper
2. 1 tbsp. all-purpose flour
3. 4 pieces boneless chicken
4. 1 tbsp. unsalted butter
5. ½ medium lemon
6. 1 cup chicken broth

NUTRITION INFORMATION

Fat	6g
Saturated Fat	2g
Carbohydrates	2g
Protein	20g
Sugar	0g

INSTRUCTIONS:
1. Take a large plate and combine lemon pepper seasoning with flour. Cover chicken with flour mixture. Heat butter on a skillet and heat chicken for about 3 minutes a side.
2. Mix lemon zest and juice with broth and pour over chicken to cook for 15min with lid. Remove lid and cook for 5 min more.

TUNA SALAD

SERVING SIZE: 1
SERVINGS PER RECIPE: 4
SMART POINTS PER SERVING: 3
CALORIES: 137
PREPARATION TIME: 10 MINUTES
INGREDIENTS:
1. 12 canned chunk white tuna
2. ½ cup celery
3. 2 tbsp. parsley and mayonnaise
4. ½ tbsp. mustard and salt
5. ¼ tbsp. black pepper

NUTRITION INFORMATION

Fat	5g
Saturated Fat	1g
Carbohydrates	1g
Protein	20g
Sugar	1g

INSTRUCTIONS:
1. Mix parsley, tuna, and celery in a bowl. Add mayonnaise, mustard, salt and pepper, and stir.

TURKEY SAUSAGE WITH BELL PEPPERS

SERVING SIZE: 1
SERVINGS PER RECIPE: 4
SMART POINTS PER SERVING: 3
CALORIES: 93
PREPARATION TIME: 25 MINUTES
INGREDIENTS:
1. 1/4lb turkey sausage
2. 1 red, yellow, green bell pepper and onion
3. ¼ cup chicken broth
4. 2 tbsp. garlic
5. 1/4 tbsp. red pepper flakes and dried oregano

NUTRITION INFORMATION

Fat	3g
Saturated Fat	0g
Carbohydrates	12g
Protein	6g
Sugar	4g

INSTRUCTIONS:
1. Heat skillet after spraying pan cooking spray.
2. Add sausage and stir for 6 min and add bell peppers, broth, onion, pepper flakes, and oregano.
3. Sauté for 5 min and heat at a simmer with lid covered for 5 min more.

CHICKEN FRIED RICE

SERVING SIZE: 1
SERVINGS PER RECIPE: 6
SMART POINTS PER SERVING: 4
CALORIES: 179
PREPARATION TIME: 25 MINUTES
INGREDIENTS:

1. 4 egg white
2. ½ cup scallion, green and white parts
3. 2 garlic cloves
4. Chopped boneless chicken
5. ½ cup carrot and frozen green peas
6. 2 cup cooked brown rice
7. 3 tbsp. soy sauce

NUTRITION INFORMATION

Fat	2g
Saturated Fat	0g
Carbohydrates	21g
Protein	18g
Sugar	2g

INSTRUCTIONS:

1. Spray the pan with cooking spray and set the pan over medium-high heat. Add egg whites and cook for 5 minutes. Remove from pan.
2. Repeat the same process to heat the pan and add scallions and garlic and sauté for 2 min. Add chicken and sauté for 15 min.
3. Mix cooked egg whites and brown rice, peas, and soy sauce. Cook until heated through.

CHICKEN AND DUMPLINGS

SERVING SIZE: 1
SERVINGS PER RECIPE: 8
SMART POINTS PER SERVING: 4
CALORIES: 105
PREPARATION TIME: 55 MINUTES
INGREDIENTS:
1. 2 can chicken broth, low fat cream of chicken soup
2. 3 cup chopped and cooked chicken breast
3. ½ tbsp. celery salt
4. salt and black pepper, to taste
5. fat-free tortillas

NUTRITION INFORMATION

Fat	4g
Saturated Fat	1g
Carbohydrates	0g
Protein	16g
Sugar	0g

INSTRUCTIONS:
1. Take a large saucepan and add chicken broth, cream of chicken soup and chicken breast, and boil it. Sprinkle salt, celery salt, and pepper.
2. Add tortillas slowly one at a time when liquid is boiling. Reduce heat and simmer for 25 min.

CHEESY EGGPLANT CASSEROLE

SERVING SIZE: 1
SERVINGS PER RECIPE: 4
SMART POINTS PER SERVING: 4
CALORIES: 79
PREPARATION TIME: 45 MINUTES
INGREDIENTS:
1. 1 cup spaghetti sauce
2. ¾ cup mozzarella cheese, cottage cheese
3. 2 tbsp. parmesan cheese
4. ¾lb eggplant

NUTRITION INFORMATION

Fat	2g
Saturated Fat	1g
Carbohydrates	11g
Protein	5g
Sugar	5g

INSTRUCTIONS:
1. Grill eggplants for 10 minutes. Spray 8x8 baking pan with nonstick spray. Put eggplant in the pan and spread spaghetti sauce over. Mix mozzarella and cottage cheese over sauce and sprinkle parmesan cheese.
2. Bake at 35 degrees for 35 minutes.

SALSA CHICKEN

SERVING SIZE: 1
SERVINGS PER RECIPE: 4
SMART POINTS PER SERVING: 4
CALORIES: 238
PREPARATION TIME: 45 MINUTES
INGREDIENTS:
1. 4 pieces boneless chicken
2. ¾ cup salsa
3. ½ cup green onion
4. ¼ cup parmesan cheese

NUTRITION INFORMATION

Fat	6g
Saturated Fat	2g
Carbohydrates	4g
Protein	40g
Sugar	2g

INSTRUCTIONS:
1. Preheat oven to 350 degrees F.
2. Place chicken in baking dish with cooking spray. Spoon salsa over chicken, top with green onions and sprinkle cheese.
3. Cover and bake for 30min.
4. Uncover and bake for 10min more.

TURKEY MEATBALLS

SERVING SIZE: 1
SERVINGS PER RECIPE: 4
SMART POINTS PER SERVING: 4
CALORIES: 200
PREPARATION TIME: 30 MINUTES
INGREDIENTS:

1. 1 lb turkey breast
2. ½ green bell pepper
3. 4 scallion
4. ⅓ cup bread crumbs
5. 1 egg white
6. 1 tbsp. soy sauce
7. 1/4 cup sweet and sour sauce
8. 1/2 cup applesauce

NUTRITION INFORMATION

Fat	1g
Saturated Fat	0g
Carbohydrates	15g
Protein	31g
Sugar	6g

INSTRUCTIONS:

1. Preheat oven to 375 degrees F and spray a pan with cooking spray.
2. Mix turkey, pepper, scallions, breadcrumbs, egg white, and soy sauce. Shape them into balls and place them in the pan. Bake for 20 minutes.
3. Mix sweet and sour sauce with applesauce. Microwave for 2min.
4. Stir the meatballs into the sauce to serve.

SALISBURY STEAK

SERVING SIZE: 1
SERVINGS PER RECIPE: 4
SMART POINTS PER SERVING: 5
CALORIES: 225
PREPARATION TIME: MINUTES
INGREDIENTS:

1. 1lb ground beef
2. ¼ tbsp. garlic powder and black pepper
3. ½ tbsp. kosher salt
4. 8 mushrooms
5. ¼ cup onion
6. 1 tbsp. dried thyme
7. 2 tbsp. dry sherry
8. 1 jar beef gravy

NUTRITION INFORMATION

Fat	8g
Saturated Fat	4g
Carbohydrates	8g
Protein	29g
Sugar	2g

INSTRUCTIONS:

1. Mix well ground beef, garlic powder, salt, and pepper. Shape them into thick patties.
2. Take a large skillet and spray cooking spray, place over medium heat until hot. Add patties and cook for 4 min.
3. Increase heat and add mushrooms, onion, and thyme; and sauté for 3min. Add sherry, sauté 1min, stir in gravy and add patties and cook for 2min.

COLA CHICKEN

SERVING SIZE: 1
SERVINGS PER RECIPE: 4
SMART POINTS PER SERVING: 5
CALORIES: 193
PREPARATION TIME: 65 MINUTES
INGREDIENTS:
1. 4 pieces of boneless chicken
2. 1 cup ketchup
3. 1 diet cola
4. ½ cup onion

NUTRITION INFORMATION

Fat	3g
Saturated Fat	1g
Carbohydrates	15g
Protein	26g
Sugar	14g

INSTRUCTIONS:
1. In skillet, mix ketchup and cola and add chicken and onions.
2. Boil and cover. Reduce heat to medium and cook for 45min.
3. Remove lid and simmer till thickens.

DINNER RECIPES

JALAPENO CHICKEN

SERVING SIZE: 1
SERVINGS PER RECIPE: 4
SMART POINTS PER SERVING: 5
CALORIES: 202
PREPARATION TIME: 15 MINUTES
INGREDIENTS:
1. 1/3 cup steak sauce
2. 1/3 cup jalapeno jelly
3. 2 tbsp. Worcestershire sauce
4. 1 tbsp. garlic powder
5. 4 pieces boneless chicken

NUTRITION INFORMATION

Fat	1g
Saturated Fat	0g
Carbohydrates	20g
Protein	26g
Sugar	15g

INSTRUCTIONS:
1. Take a large plastic bag and add steak sauce, jalapeno jelly, Worcestershire sauce, and garlic powder. Add chicken to the bag and shake till the chicken is coated. Marinate for 8 hours minimum turning the bag occasionally.
2. Remove the chicken from bag. Coat a grill rack with cooking spray and place it over medium-hot coals about 400 degrees F. Grill the chicken for 5 min each side.

CHICKEN NOODLE SOUP

SERVING SIZE: 1
SERVINGS PER RECIPE: 4
SMART POINTS PER SERVING: 5
CALORIES: 170
PREPARATION TIME: 30 MINUTES
INGREDIENTS:

1. 8 oz chicken breast
2. 5 cup chicken broth
3. 1 cup thin spaghetti
4. ½ cup carrots and celery
5. 8 green onion
6. ¼ tbsp. dried thyme and parsley
7. Salt and black pepper to taste

NUTRITION INFORMATION

Fat	2g
Saturated Fat	0g
Carbohydrates	10g
Protein	26g
Sugar	0g

INSTRUCTIONS:

1. Season chicken with salt and black pepper. Heat a skillet over medium-high heat and spray cooking spray. Add chicken and cook for 5 minutes stirring constantly.
2. Add chicken broth, spaghetti, carrots, celery, green onion, thyme, parsley, and chicken soup in a pot. Boil on reduce heat and simmer spaghetti.

CROCKPOT CHICKEN CHILI

SERVING SIZE: 1
SERVINGS PER RECIPE: 8
SMART POINTS PER SERVING: 5
CALORIES: 160
PREPARATION TIME: 490 MINUTES
INGREDIENTS:
1. 12 oz boneless chicken
2. 1 envelope chili seasoning mix
3. 1 qt canned tomatoes
4. 1 can corn and kidney beans
5. 1 green bell pepper and onion
6. ½ cup salsa

NUTRITION INFORMATION

Fat	2g
Saturated Fat	0g
Carbohydrates	24g
Protein	14g
Sugar	7g

INSTRUCTIONS:
1. Sear the chicken in a nonstick skillet coated with cooking spray.
2. To a crock pot add chicken, chili seasoning mix, tomatoes, kidney beans, bell pepper, onion, and salsa.
3. Cover and cook on low for 7 hours.

BALSAMIC CHICKEN

SERVING SIZE: 1
SERVINGS PER RECIPE: 4
SMART POINTS PER SERVING: 5
CALORIES: 193
PREPARATION TIME: 30 MINUTES
INGREDIENTS:
1. 3 pieces of boneless chicken
2. Salt and black pepper to taste
3. ¼ cup all-purpose flour
4. 2/3 cup chicken broth
5. 1 ½ tbsp. cornstarch
6. ½ cup raspberry preserves
7. 1 ½ tbsp. balsamic vinegar

NUTRITION INFORMATION

Fat	10g
Saturated Fat	2g
Carbohydrates	32g
Protein	26g
Sugar	5g

INSTRUCTIONS:
1. Season chicken with salt and pepper. Cover the chicken with flour completely.
2. Cook chicken in skillet for 15 min on medium heat, turning halfway through.
3. Remove chicken from skillet. Add chicken broth, cornstarch, and raspberry preserve in skillet and heat at medium. Stir in balsamic vinegar. Add back the chicken and cook for 10 min, turning halfway through.

CRUMBED BAKED CHICKEN

SERVING SIZE: 1
SERVINGS PER RECIPE: 4
SMART POINTS PER SERVING: 5
CALORIES: 194
PREPARATION TIME: 55 MINUTES
INGREDIENTS:
1. 2 tbsp. orange juice and Dijon mustard
2. ¼ tbsp. salt
3. ¾ cup whole-wheat crackers
4. 1 tbsp. orange zest
5. 1 shallot
6. ¼ tbsp. black paper
7. 12 oz boneless chicken thigh

NUTRITION INFORMATION

Fat	7g
Saturated Fat	2g
Carbohydrates	15g
Protein	19g
Sugar	1g

INSTRUCTIONS:
1. Preheat oven to 350 degrees F.
2. Take a bowl and combine orange juice, mustard, and salt. Combine the cracker crumbs, orange zest, shallot, and pepper on a sheet of wax paper. Apply mustard on both sides of chicken and mix it with crumbs.
3. Bake 15 minutes, turn over, and bake till cooked through.

CRAB QUESADILLAS

SERVING SIZE: 1
SERVINGS PER RECIPE: 4
SMART POINTS PER SERVING: 9
CALORIES: 290
PREPARATION TIME: 20 MINUTES
INGREDIENTS:

1. 8 oz imitation crabmeat
2. ½ cup cheddar cheese
3. 1 can green chili
4. ¼ cup tomato
5. 2 tbsp. green bell pepper
6. 4 tortillas

NUTRITION INFORMATION

Fat	9g
Saturated Fat	4g
Carbohydrates	39g
Protein	13g
Sugar	6g

INSTRUCTIONS:

1. Preheat oven at 425 degrees F.
2. Take a bowl and mix crabmeat, cheese, chilies, tomatoes, and bell pepper.
3. Spray a cooking spray on one side of the tortilla. Turn it over and put crab mixture on the unsprayed portion and fold.
4. Place quesadilla on a baking sheet. Bake for 10 minutes and turn over and bake for 5 minutes more.

QUICK CHILI

SERVING SIZE: 1
SERVINGS PER RECIPE: 6
SMART POINTS PER SERVING: 7
CALORIES: 278
PREPARATION TIME: 20 MINUTES
INGREDIENTS:
1. 1 lb ground beef or turkey
2. 1 onion and clove garlic
3. 1 ½ cup water
4. 1 tbsp. chili powder
5. 1 tbsp. salt
6. 16 oz canned chili beans
7. 6 oz can tomato paste

NUTRITION INFORMATION

Fat	8g
Saturated Fat	3g
Carbohydrates	28g
Protein	24g
Sugar	4g

INSTRUCTIONS:
1. Take a large saucepan and cook meat, onion, and garlic on medium high heat.
2. Drain in colander and then rinse it with warm water, and then return to pan.
3. Cover and reduce heat. Simmer for 15 min.

CILANTRO AND LIME SHRIMP

SERVING SIZE: 1
SERVINGS PER RECIPE: 4
SMART POINTS PER SERVING: 3
CALORIES: 177
PREPARATION TIME: 20 MINUTES
INGREDIENTS:
1. 1 ¾ lb shrimp
2. ½ tbsp. ground cumin and salt
3. 2 tbsp. lime juice
4. ¼ tbsp. ground ginger and pepper
5. 2 garlic cloves
6. 1 tbsp. olive oil
7. ¼ cup cilantro
8. 1 tbsp. lime

NUTRITION INFORMATION

Fat	6g
Saturated Fat	1g
Carbohydrates	3g
Protein	27g
Sugar	0g

INSTRUCTIONS:
1. Take a bowl, combine shrimp, lime juice, cumin, ginger and garlic, and toss well.
2. In a skillet, heat oil over medium-high heat. Add shrimp mixture and sauté for 4 min.
3. Stop heating and stir in cilantro, lime zest, salt and pepper.

CHICKEN AND CHEESE CASSEROLE

SERVING SIZE: 1
SERVINGS PER RECIPE: 8
SMART POINTS PER SERVING: 5
CALORIES: 153
PREPARATION TIME: 55 MINUTES
INGREDIENTS:
1. 2 cup macaroni, boneless chicken, skim milk, and cream of mushroom soup
2. 8 oz cheddar cheese

NUTRITION INFORMATION

Fat	4g
Saturated Fat	2g
Carbohydrates	16g
Protein	12g
Sugar	1g

INSTRUCTIONS:
1. Preheat oven to 350 degrees F.
2. Take a casserole dish and mix macaroni, chicken, cream of mushroom soup, skim milk, and cheddar cheese. Mix well.
3. Cover and bake for 45 min.
4. Remove cover and bake for 15 min.

BARBECUE MEATLOAF

SERVING SIZE: 1
SERVINGS PER RECIPE: 4
SMART POINTS PER SERVING: 7
CALORIES: 240
PREPARATION TIME: 45 MINUTES
INGREDIENTS:
1. 1 lb ground beef
2. ½ cup barbecue sauce
3. ¼ cup frozen onion
4. ¼ cup bread crumbs
5. 2 egg white

NUTRITION INFORMATION

Fat	6g
Saturated Fat	3g
Carbohydrates	17g
Protein	27g
Sugar	9g

INSTRUCTIONS:
1. Preheat oven to 375 degrees F.
2. Take a large bowl, combine meat, barbecue sauce, onion, bread crumbs, and egg whites; and stir well.
3. Shape mixture into a loaf and spread barbecue sauce over it.
4. Bake at 375 degrees F for 40 minutes.

TUNA PASTA SALAD

SERVING SIZE: 1
SERVINGS PER RECIPE: 6
SMART POINTS PER SERVING: 5
CALORIES: 194
PREPARATION TIME: 25 MINUTES
INGREDIENTS:
1. 6 oz pasta
2. 1 can tuna in water
3. ½ cup yellow bell pepper, cherry tomato
4. ¼ cup celery
5. ¾ cup salsa
6. ½ cup mayonnaise
7. ½ tbsp. red pepper
8. 2 tbsp. scallion

NUTRITION INFORMATION

Fat	2g
Saturated Fat	1g
Carbohydrates	25g
Protein	18g
Sugar	2g

INSTRUCTIONS:
1. Cook pasta according to the package direction, skipping salt and fat
2. Drain pasta, rinse in cold water, and drain again
3. Take a large bowl, combine pasta, tuna, bell pepper, cherry tomatoes, and celery.
4. Take a small bowl, combine salsa, mayonnaise, and red pepper. Sprinkle with scallions.

STIR FRIED CHINESE VEGETABLES

SERVING SIZE: 1
SERVINGS PER RECIPE: 4
SMART POINTS PER SERVING: 1
CALORIES: 42
PREPARATION TIME: 12 MINUTES
INGREDIENTS:
1. ¼ cup chicken broth
2. 1 tbsp. low-sodium soy sauce
3. 2 garlic cloves minced
4. 1 ½ tbsp. fresh ginger peeled and minced
5. 2 cups bok Choy, chopped
6. 1 red bell pepper seeded and cut
7. 1 cup snow peas
8. ½ carrots sliced
9. ¼ cups sliced bamboo shoots
10. ¼ cups sliced water chestnuts

NUTRITION INFORMATION

Fat	0 g
Saturated Fat	0 g
Carbohydrates	8 g
Protein	3 g
Sugar	4 g

INSTRUCTIONS:
1. Mix chicken broth, soy sauce, ginger and garlic in a bowl.
2. Heat the oil in a large skillet. Fry bok Choy and bell pepper for 3 minutes. Add the above broth mixture, snow peas, and carrot. Reduce the heat and cook for about 3 minutes till sauce thickens and vegetables become tender.
3. Stir in bamboo shoots and water chestnuts for about 1 minute.

PITA PIZZA

SERVING SIZE: 1
SERVINGS PER RECIPE: 1
SMART POINTS PER SERVING: 9
CALORIES: 341
PREPARATION TIME: 12 MINUTES
INGREDIENTS:
1. 1 large thin pita bread
2. ¼ cup pizza sauce
3. ¼ cup mushrooms
4. ¼ cup green pepper
5. 10 small black olives
6. ½ cup fat-free mozzarella cheese
7. 2 tbsp. parmesan cheese
8. A pinch of pizza seasoning

NUTRITION INFORMATION

Fat	6 g
Saturated Fat	1 g
Carbohydrates	45 g
Protein	27 g
Sugar	4 g

INSTRUCTIONS:
1. Preheat the oven.
2. Spread pizza sauce on the bread. First layer the vegetables. Top with mozzarella, parmesan, and pizza seasoning.
3. Spray a cooking spray over the cheese.
4. Put in the oven for about 2 minutes until the cheese is melted.

BLT PASTA SALAD

SERVING SIZE: 1
SERVINGS PER RECIPE: 6
SMART POINTS PER SERVING: 7
CALORIES: 86
PREPARATION TIME: 15 MINUTES
INGREDIENTS:

1. 3 cups large macaroni shells pasta, cooked
2. 4 cups tomatoes
3. 4 slices cooked bacon
4. 3 cups lettuce
5. 1 tbsp. sugar
6. 2 tbsp. cider vinegar
7. ½ cup fat-free mayonnaise
8. ¼ cup sour cream
9. 1 tbsp. Dijon mustard
10. Salt and pepper to taste

NUTRITION INFORMATION

Fat	5 g
Saturated Fat	2 g
Carbohydrates	10 g
Protein	6 g
Sugar	3 g

INSTRUCTIONS:

1. Mix pasta, bacon, tomatoes, and lettuce in a bowl.
2. Mix sugar, vinegar, mayonnaise, sour cream, and mustard in a bowl. Add salt and pepper accordingly.
3. Pour dressing over the pasta mixture, stir to combine and chill. Serve.

EGG SALAD

SERVING SIZE: 1
SERVINGS PER RECIPE: 4
SMART POINTS PER SERVING: 3
CALORIES: 106
PREPARATION TIME: 20 MINUTES
INGREDIENTS:

1. 4 eggs.
2. 2 eggs boiled egg whites. Remove the yolk from whole eggs after boiling
3. 2 tbsp. fresh chives
4. 2 tbsp. mayonnaise
5. ½ tbsp. Dijon mustard
6. Salt to taste
7. Dill
8. ¼ tbsp. black pepper

NUTRITION INFORMATION

Fat	7 g
Saturated Fat	2 g
Carbohydrates	1 g
Protein	8 g
Sugar	1 g

INSTRUCTIONS:

1. Place eggs in a saucepan and boil them.
2. Remove shells when they are cooled.
3. Discard yolk from 2 of the eggs. Cut the remaining eggs and egg whites.
4. Transfer eggs to another bowl. Add chives, mustard, mayonnaise, dill, salt, and pepper. Blend the mixture.

CHICKEN SALAD

SERVING SIZE: 1
SERVINGS PER RECIPE: 4
SMART POINTS PER SERVING: 4
CALORIES: 195
PREPARATION TIME: 20 MINUTES
INGREDIENTS:

1. 1 lb boneless, skinless chicken breast
2. ½ cup celery
3. ¼ cup dill pickle
4. ¼ cup mayonnaise
5. 2 tbsp. sour cream
6. 2 tbsp. parsley
7. 1 tbsp. Dijon mustard
8. 1 tbsp. lemon juice
9. Salt and pepper

NUTRITION INFORMATION

Fat	9 g
Saturated Fat	2 g
Carbohydrates	3 g
Protein	25 g
Sugar	1 g

INSTRUCTIONS:

1. Place chicken in a saucepan and bring to a boil. Drain the water. Cut the chicken after it is cool.
2. Put the chicken in a bowl and add celery, mayonnaise, sour cream, parsley, mustard, pickles, lemon juice, salt, and pepper. Mix until blended.

ABOUT THE AUTHOR

James Houck is a health and fitness enthusiast who loves teaching people about healthy ways to lose weight and live the best life they can.

Over the years, he has studied what works and what doesn't in health and fitness. He is passionate about helping others achieve great success in their diet and exercise endeavor through his books and seminars.

His biggest satisfaction is when he finds out that he was able to help someone attain the results they've been looking for. In his free time, he loves to spend time with his 2-year-old daughter.

39688361R00036

Made in the USA
Middletown, DE
22 January 2017